I0428456

Restore Your Vision in 9 Easy Ways

Michel Lee

DEDICATION

This book is dedicated to the Bates method and the accommodation principle which prove that vision loss is repairable and good and healthy vision can be restored and eye glasses dropped through eye exercises and healthy habits.

CONTENTS

1 INTRODUCTION

Thank you for buying this book! I have worn glasses since I was four years old. It has been my life long quest to get rid of my glasses and to improve my vision.

I sincerely hope that you will be able to restore eye sight, the most wonderful and precious gift to mankind.

In the 2nd chapter I tell you about the structure of the human eyes.

The 3rd to the 11th chapters are the nine ways which will help you a lot in restoring your vision, however you must do them diligently.

In the 12th chapter I tell you a daily regimen which will help you in keeping eyes healthy.

Lastly I give tips to maintain and restore eyesight.

2 HUMAN EYES

Understand the Eye

"The eye sees a thing more clearly in dreams than the imagination awake." – Leonardo da Vinci

Eyes are the most wonderful gift to the man and yet the most neglected part. This is due to the addiction of people with computers, TV, gadgets, tablets and part due to the speed of life which has increased, which has led the modern man to become restless, anxious and worrisome. No more the modern man takes out time to take leisurely walks, enjoy the simple things like life like gardening, taking life easily. The result is that the gift of eyes which used to last for a 100 years now lasts much less. Man has learnt about the sciences, medicine, made great progress but little does he know about himself, And even lesser discipline he has now. As you go through this book this book will advice you not only how you can treat the condition but also will try to make you aware of the causes which led to this condition.

Let us first look at the structure of the eye in order to increase our insight into the eye. This book will assume that the reader is a layman and will offer advice as such.

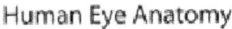

Human Eye Anatomy

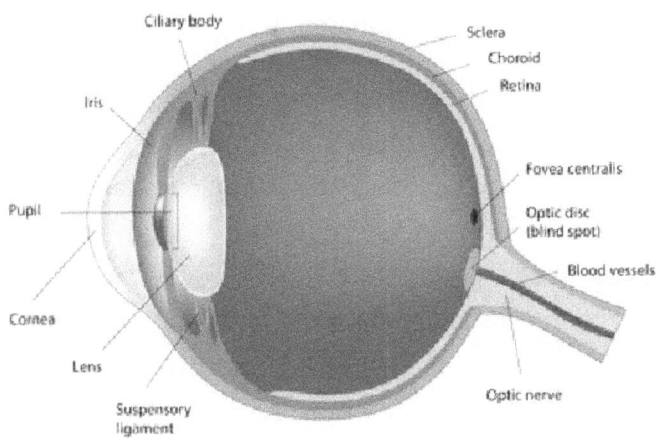

Ciliary Body – This is the circumferential tissue inside the eye composed of ciliary muscles (which cause accommodation similar to the lens of a camera). It changes the shape of the lens within the eye.

Iris - Iris is a thin circular structure in the eye. It is responsible for controlling the diameter and size of the pupils and thus the amount of light reaching the retina.

The iris consists of two layers the stroma (consisting of fiber and cells) and beneath the stroma pigmented epithelial cells.

Pupil – The pupil is a hole located in the center of the iris which allows the light to enter.

Cornea – The transparent front part of the eye covering iris, pupil and anterior chamber. It does not have blood vessels as they would impair transparency. It receives nutrients from the diffusion of the tear fluids. It receives oxygen directly from the air. Oxygen first dissolves in the tears and then diffuses throughout the cornea to keep it healthy. The human cornea has five layers.

Lens – It is a transparent, biconvex structure in the eye, that along with cornea helps to reflect light to focus it on the retina.

The adjustment of the lens in order to convey a sharp image on the retina is called accommodation and this is procedure is similar to the lens of a photographic camera.

Water soluble proteins account for over 90% of the composition of the lens. The lens is comprised of three main parts lens capsule, the lens epithelium and the lens fibers. Glucose is the primary energy source of the lens. Cataract is opacity of the lens.

Suspensory Ligament – This is a ligament which prevents the downward displacement of the eye.

Optic Nerve – It transmits the visual information from the retina to the brain. It is composed of retinal ganglion cell axons and support cells. Each human optic nerve contains between 770,000 and 1.7 million nerve fibers.

Blood Vessels – These are part of the circulatory system which transports blood to the entire body. Oxygen bound to the hemoglobin in red blood cells is the most critical nutrient carried by the blood. They play a huge role in virtually every medical condition.

Optic Disk – This is the entry point for the major blood vessels that supply the retina.

Fovea Centralis – It is responsible for the sharp central vision.

Retina – It is a light sensitive tissue, when light strikes it, it initiates a cascade of chemical and electrical events that ultimately trigger nerve impulses.

Choroid – It provides oxygen and nourishment to the outer layers of the retina

Sclera – Also known as the white of the eye. It is opaque, fibrous, protective layer of the eye containing collagen and elastic fiber.

Factors which can increase the risk of vision problems

- Smoking

- Air pollution

- Alcohol consumption

- Medicine side effects

- High salt intake

- High sugar intake

- Exposure to UV

- Exposure to radiation

- Stress

- Hypertension

- Improper nutrition

- Eye Strain

- Viewing electronic displays for long durations

- Tranquilizers

- Low Vitamin A diet

- High Dairy products intake

3 BREATHING RIGHT

Breathing is the most important function of the human body. Almost all other functions depend on it. Man most of the time breathes incorrectly either due to clothing which restricts the breathing like tight jeans or pants with belt or due to stress, or plainly just incorrect habits of breathing. Done properly this could lead to vitality of the human body, help the man in keeping the degenerative diseases and old age at bay and done wrongly it leads to the fast progress of old age and degenerative diseases of the eyes. If you can take just this one fact out of the book and incorporate it into your life this book would have served its purpose. Learning to breathe is a science and this small chapter may not do complete justice to It but you will take the first steps.

Babies do something better than people, they naturally know how to breathe right through the belly. If you see a baby breath you will see his belly going up and down, in a rhythmic fashion and calm composed breaths. How many of us have do this right a very small percentage. When we worry, fret over things, hurry, get angry during the day our breathing corresponds it. For a day notice how you breathe when you feel ecstatic on seeing someone you love and when you worry and fret. Once your emotions take a dive down your breathing corresponds and it becomes a vicious cycle.

There are multiple types of breathing; primarily you can breathe through the chest or through the belly or both. Breathing through the belly and through chest can be called a complete breath. And this we will use in our quest to beat the progress of the degenerative eye diseases. You need to fill up your body with oxygen, the extra oxygen will cleanse the blood, provide energy to the body and flush out toxins. During the day you need to follow the following approach listed in the following paragraphs.

When you wake up in the morning you need to go outside in fresh air. Begin to inhale several complete breaths. You need to fill up the body of oxygen to drive out the toxins, cleanse the blood, and provide energy to the body. The level of oxygen in the body can be increased in a very short time with rapid breathing. You can follow this approach or design your own. Take 20 complete breaths each breath inhalation + exhalation lasting 1 second. Then you can take 20 more complete breaths with each inhalation + exhalation lasting 2 seconds. Then you can take 20 more complete breaths with each cycle lasting 4 seconds. The entire set of 20 rapid, 20 medium and 20 long complete breaths can be repeated as long as the person feels comfortable. You can also rub your hands and do brisk walking very soon when the bodies' oxygen level rises you may start to feel tingling sensation in different parts of your body. This is normal. You should stop when you start feeling uneasy or uncomfortable. This process will also make you thirsty and you should drink water after completing this.

During the day while you are work or in the evening when you relax remember to keep taking complete breaths. This will keep your body charged the whole day as well as keep you in a good mood and beat stress. This will also prevent the degenerative disease from causing harm. Make sure that your nostrils remain clear and you do not breathe from the mouth. If you find yourself breathing from the mouth because you can't breathe normally through nostrils then close each nostril one by one and breathe through a single nostril. Once this is done most often you would be able to breathe normally. If you still can't breathe normally go to a restroom and wash your nostrils with water.

Taking complete breaths throughout the day will ensure that you get sufficient energy during the day and the degenerative diseases find it hard to progress. The Pranayams is an efficient and important set of exercises which help the body to fight against any illness naturally.

4 WALKING

Walking is considered very good for health. There are several reasons for it. The soles of the feet have acupressure points which get pressed when you walk. However real benefit only takes place when you walk at leisure and not when you walk at work or at home. You need to ensure that you take a leisurely walk in the early morning or evening, wearing jogging suit and jogging shoes. You need to practice walking in exactly the same way I am telling you to beat this disease.

Combine complete breathing which I have told you in the earlier section when you walk. Remember to complete sets of long, medium and short breaths as already taught. Walk briskly and also at times rub your hands against each other, through the thumbs of your hand press against the palm of your other hand. Make sure you press your hands together for a good amount of time at the same time keep taking complete breaths.

During the day when you get a chance to go for lunch count your steps to and back from the eating joint. If you do not go outside to eat after you have lunch take a walk outside and count at least 200 steps. If you forget begin counting each step from 1. This is a very easy approach to keep the mind off from worries and thoughts. This will make your eyes see more and you will notice that you will see a number of things on the way which you did not see before. Also as you see several objects try to see them crisply. If you see greenery try to focus your eyes on it and see it. The simple process of watching the objects will exercise your eyes and help your vision. It will also stop the eye diseases from progressing and will restore your vision.

5 HEALTHY EATING HABITS

It doesn't take rocket science to understand that we become what we eat. The moment you start eating healthy it slowly affects you in a positive way. Although it is not noticeable but over a short period of time you can feel the difference. If your eyes are stressed and you feel uneasy eat an apple and see how different your eyes feel after it. You also need to watch out for a number of foods that will harm you in this condition. In the following paragraphs I will discuss the foods that harm you and the foods that help you. Combing the process of breathing right, walking and eating will yield you tremendous results.

Let me begin with the foods that will harm you. If you are a regular drinker of milk or coffee you need to cut down on it. You need to cut down on sugary drinks, colas, chocolate and snack foods. You need to stop alcohol consumption and stop smoking. Alcohol and smoking can cause cataract in your eyes. If you already have cataract they are a poison that you would rather keep at bay. Also beware of passive smoke. When you encounter such a situation walk out or away from the nearby smoker. Cataract can progress rapidly if the eyes come in touch of cigarette smoke.

There are a number of foods that will help your eyes a lot. Primarily carrots, freshly squeezed pineapple juice, bilberries and blueberries, antioxidant rich food, green vegetables and fruits. Through the day eat a lot of green vegetables and fruits if you are not in the habit of eating them increase your diet and eat healthy. Cut down on potato chips, snacks, colas, and junk food like pizza. When you already are in the grips of eye disease you need to be very cautious of what you eat. You need to be disciplined without discipline nothing can be achieved. You need to follow a system and form habits, if you do not form a habit of eating right, and occasionally skip from your plan so will the degenerative disease start and make your condition worse.

Remember to drink lot of fluids in the form of water, lime juice or fresh fruit juices. Processed fruit juices and sliced or cut fruit that you buy from the store also has lost about 80% of its nutritious value. You need to take fresh fruit juice which has been squeezed within half an hour to get full benefit. This also needs to be done routinely to help the body keep up its fight.

6 WATER THERAPY

The process of water therapy is simple when you wake up in the morning drink 5 glasses of water before you eat or drink any other thing. Doing this consistently for months people have dissolved kidney stones. This is a very simple process and yet so hard to follow. It is difficult to drink 5 glasses of water after you wake up. In the beginning you may not feel like it but you can slowly increase the number of glasses of water you drink. Say for example the first week when you wake you can take 1 glass of water, then the next week you can begin to take 2 until you reach the daily 5 glasses of water. You will urinate a lot due to this but harmful toxins which are in your body will get flushed out.

You cannot drink 2-3 glass of water in the morning and then intake a couple more after 1 or 2 hours. This will not work. You need to intake 5 glasses of water when you wake up within half an hour to make this process effective.

7 ANTIOXIDANTS

You need to take sufficient amounts of antioxidants during the day to inhibit the diseases. There are a number of books written on the foods that have a rich amount of antioxidants. Antioxidants help the body and will help restoring the vision problems because they limit the effect of body processes that cause the body to age. See an apple that has gone bad. When an apple has gone bad there are several processes that will occur to cause it to rot faster. These are the same processes that will cause the degenerative diseases of the eyes.

During the day take sufficient amount of green tea, fresh fruits and fresh vegetables. Fresh corn has a lot of antioxidants and vitamins which help the eyes. You can refer to books on the internet which will detail you on this.

8 YOGA

There are a number of different yogas which help in restoring vision disorders. In the coming paragraph I will detail you the yogas that will help you in this condition. You need to make sure that you do this as a routine and do It daily to help the body over the long term. Remember anything not done routinely as a habit would not be effective enough, I am iterating this again so that you remember the significance of this.

The first yoga that I want to tell you is the Surya Namaskar. You need to research the details of this yoga on your own. The yoga in itself is very simple it comprises of 12 postures that you need to do in a flow. I will tell you about the significance of this yoga philosophically. Surya means the Sun. Sun is considered to be a constant. Being like the sun is being full of energy and life, in this condition no disease can take root and progress in the body. When you worship the sun by doing this yoga imagine that you are receiving the sun's blessing to have a healthy energetic body and the diseases are flowing out of the system. This yoga done at least 4 times a day will ensure that the vision problems remains at bay.

The other yogas that I want to tell you about are the Pranayams. Pranayams are also yoga and they are a set of exercises which you can do through breathing. The most beneficial Pranayams for cataract is AnulomVilom and Kalpabhatti. In AnulomVilom Pranayam you take turns and breath through the other nostril. You can get the details from the internet on how to do this, I will detail you on the philosophical aspect of this yoga. The right nostril is related to sun and the left nostril the moon. During the day without your notice you will breathe either through the left or the right nostril. This is normal. The health benefits of doing this can be realized instantly.

The other important yoga for vision problems is Kalpabhatti. The name of this yoga means that a person practicing this yoga will have a shining forehead. This yoga benefits the eyes a lot. The philosophical aspect of Kalpabhatti Pranayam is that it will raise the life's essence present in your lower chakras of the body to the head. Once this essence rises it will help in keeping the degenerative diseases of the eyes at bay.

9 STRESS REDUCTION

If you have constantly bad humour your risk of getting vision problems rises. This also means stress because bad humour and stress go hand in hand. So what are the tools to beat the stress from your daily life? I have already detailed you a powerful theory of complete breaths. When you begin to follow this approach you will almost immediately see that stress has vanished from your day. You can begin to live a stress free life. Saying it for me is easy because I have practiced it and seen the effect of it in my daily life. It works for me, several of my followers and will work for you too.

There are a number of ways to beat stress. Whatever the level of stress you can beat it. Even if you are in a prison cell you can follow the methods that I will hint in the coming paragraphs and you will be able to succeed in keeping yourself calm and stress free.

Do I really mean what I have said earlier? Yes. I will detail you the power of transcendental meditation. When you combine what I have taught you so far and include transcendental meditation in the set of exercises you can beat the demon of stress. I will only hint at this process in this manual and will leave it to you to unfold its complete possibilities.

This kind of meditation is the core of religions which I believe. When a person is deep in the process of praying the harmful chemicals do not get released in the brain which get released normally when a person is angry, stressed or feeling resentful. Instead of harmful chemicals protective chemicals and energy is emitted which heals. This fact is not recognized by the medical science but I and so many other followers of religion have found this to be true. This is why so many religions exist because the power of prayer does work. It does cause magic. Anything without substance cannot survive.

Imagine a scenario if you are in stressful environment and there is a person who likes to take jabs at you. Normally you would feel hurt, angry and resentful but if instead of bringing these emotions forward you meditate you have started helping yourself positively. In the end you will end up in a better situation that the person was taking pot shots at you.

To summarize if you simply take complete breaths throughout the day and remember to take complete breaths in stressful situations, stress will remain at bay. There is nothing simpler than this.

10 HUMOUR

Laughter is the best medicine and rightly so. The process of including positive humor in your life is simple. Watch comedy channels and programs that have a positive humor that you enjoy. Doing this as a routine will keep your mood refreshed, positive and you will feel positive during your days. An hour of television a day can help you to feel better in your life, provided you watch the right of programs that keep you light. You however need to watch and take care not to watch excessive television as this can cause your eyesight to go worse.

There are so much of jokes, humor on the internet which is free. Just type the word joke and you are bombarded with sites which can cater to any type of funny bone. Use it as a tool to keep yourself relaxed during the day and don't bother if the person next to you thinks that you are a jerk for laughing all by yourself. If you do not know there are laughing clubs which you can join. A club where people just laugh seems absurd right? This is because of the grim lifestyle that so many people lead starting from the morning newspaper filled with gory grim details.

I would not go into the chemical and biological detail as to what happens when you have a positive humor throughout the day but I will let you experience it yourself. I will suggest you get a funny joke book and read through it several times a day, access jokes on the internet and watch "just for laughs" kinds of programs. I have found the Mr. Beans series to be very helpful in making me laugh ☺

11 QI GONG

Qi Gong is a vast subject many books have been written on this subject, I will try to give you the essence of this. Qi Gong is based on three pillars the right body posture, the right thoughts and right breathing. I have already detailed you the complete breath. If you follow these three mindful corrections during the day you will notice that Qi will increase in your body. More Qi means less fatigue and tiredness. Wherever your thoughts go Qi goes there.

When you want to heal vision problems through Qi you need to direct your thoughts to the area of the eyes. Focus your Qi in eyes, take your fingers and rub around your eyes. There are several acupressure and acupuncture points around your eyes and if you simple just take your fingers and rub around the area of the eyes, more Qi will flow in it. While you do this also take complete breaths and make sure that the posture of your body is correct. If you have a wrong posture Qi will find it hard to pass through.

Qi Gong details a number of exercises which help. I will detail you the most basic and yet the most effective exercise which will help you beat vision problems

. Stand in the early mornings with your legs slightly bent and bring your hands close to your face with palms facing your eyes. Stand still and feel the energy of the earth passing through your body and travelling from your palms to eyes. If you do this right you will feel energized. Practice around with various exercises, postures and keep varying, unless you feel energy passing the exercise is futile and as good as not doing.

Healing Signs

When you are doing breathing exercises like Pranayam if you start feeling a tingling sensation or like a tingling sensation, this means that the eyes are getting healed. You will get this sensation when you are doing the Anulom Vilom Pranayam (This pranayam can be performed by closing from one nostril and inhaling from the other and then inhaling from the same nostril and exhaling from the other and repeating this process). Not always can you feel this sensation and you may get this sensation occasionally. For this to happen you need to make sure that your body and mind are relaxed and that your eyes are relaxed completely and your body has a high oxygen and energy level.

Once the healing starts taking place continue to do this pranayam for maximum benefit. You can also try to promote healing of the eyes and reversal of vision problems by inhaling deeply and visualizing the oxygen reaching the eyes.

Michel Lee

12 MORE TIPS FOR RESTORING VISION

1. Get plenty of exercise. This is because exercise has effect on the entire physical body and mind. Exercise helps to strengthen the body, the immune system, beats depression, causes weight loss, boosts esteem and can increase individual's sex appeal. Health care providers call exercising as the wonder drug. There is enough evidence that exercise even promotes better sleep. It is important to have a good nutritious diet in order to help aid the restoration process in the body after strenuous exercise.

Exercising does not need to be only in a Gym, you can take up a physical sport such as tennis or swimming. You can even start with simple exercises at home like sit ups and pushups. To increase the strength of the body you can follow this simple approach. First find out how many sit ups and pushups you are able to do easily. For example you are able to do 5 pushups easily. To increase the strength of the body you can perform 5 pushups then take some rest and again perform 5 pushups. Slowly and steadily you will notice that you are able to increase the amount of pushups that you can perform, there are some very good programs online which claim that you can do a 100 pushups in a go in just about 3 months or so. You can go ahead and try these programs which will increase the strength of your body.

2. Wash your eyes with a lot of water multiple times a day. The eyes are composed of about 90% water. When you flush your eyes with water it helps the eyes to relax, the tension present in the eyes is reduced and clarity of vision is increased.

When splashing the eyes with water the eyes becomes closed automatically to prevent this you can fill your mouth completely with air or water. This will prevent the eyes from closing when you are splashing the eyes with water. You can even buy eyecups online which will aid you in washing the eyes with water.

3. De-Stress. Stress is the number one silent killer, over a long period of time this stress can manifest in a number of diseases and chronic conditions. It is also known to worsen the existing condition. If you are stressed you need to find out ways in which you can reduce or eliminate your stress. Vision Problems can worsen very quickly when you are stressed.

There are various ways in which you can de stress by building relationships with people who enjoy the same hobby, walking, soothing music and more. If you are stressed at work think about ways in which you can de stress like taking a short walk, counting your breaths and repeating a motivational quote in your mind to yourself.

4. Avoid dairy products. Dairy products may increase the progression of some vision problems. Try to decrease your dairy products intake and if possible avoid taking them before sleeping. They can impair the eyes ability to clear the toxins.

5. Read the drugs side effects section. If vision is effected due to the side effects of drugs, discuss with your health care provider and get some alternatives. Using such a medicine will increase the risk of more vision problems.

6. Go to the beach. Getting a good bath at the beach is great for the overall physical and emotional health. Spend time at the beach, enjoy the waves, play in sand at the same time protect yourself with UV rays from the sun by getting a UV Blocking sun glasses.

7. Watch your breath. Watching the breath is a powerful meditation technique if you are stressed, start counting the breaths to relax; the more relaxed you are the more peaceful your breathing will be. This can be learned with practice.

8. Walks. Go for long walks in the mornings and evenings. Both these times are very beneficial for overall health of the body. Walk for about half an hour in the mornings and in the evenings. Look around see the greenery, watch every detail and focus your eyes on the various objects.

9. Exercise your eye balls. Keep the head steady and move your eye balls by watching an extreme left point and an extreme right point and switching the point every half second. Do the same by changing the points to an extreme up and extreme down point, do this as long as you are comfortable. Rotate your eye balls in circles.

10. Stop Smoking. Smoking can cause cataract in eyes and other vision problems. If you already have cataract and you smoke too, the smoking inevitably increases the progress of cataract. Stopping smoking completely is best to prevent the cataract from increasing at a rapid pace. Also try to reduce passive smoking by choosing not to walk behind a smoker or sitting near one.

11. Stop Alcohol. Alcohol abuse is also known to cause blurry vision, cataracts and more.

12. Yoga. There are a number of yoga asanas that can do good for the eyes. The progress is very slow but worth it. Yoga also has a stream of exercises related with breathing known as Pranayams, these have proven to be very effective for a number of

conditions. A number of people claim miracles by using these exercises.

13. Eyes need to be kept relaxed so they can heal themselves and keep themselves in best working condition.

14. Acupressure. Around the eye there are a number of acupressure and acupuncture points. The novice can simply press around the eyes without causing eye pain. The area around the eye that feels good when you press in a way signifies that a positive change is happening.

15. Dry eyes. Dry eyes are dry because something is blocking the tear gland, make sure that you massage around the eye over the acupressure points. Do not stay in air conditioned environment as much possible and keep washing eyes with water.

16. Make juices your daily habit. Get natural fresh pineapple juice, wheatgrass juice, carrot juice. Eat blueberries and bilberries, bilberry consumption may inhibit or reverse eye disorders such as macular degeneration.

17. Get more of antioxidants like green tea in your diet. Antioxidants are being investigated for the prevention of many diseases.

18. VITAMINS. Some vitamins can help a lot in promoting good vision like Vitamin A which maintains healthy cells in the body and is known to support vision. A daily intake of 800 to 1,000 mcg per day is recommended. Vitamin C taken daily can help reduce the chances of vision problems by up to 70 percent. Approximately 1 to 2 g of vitamin C per day is ideal. Vitamin E can help reverse the effects of free radicals and delay eye problems. The recommended daily dose of vitamin E is 15 mg. Selenium and Vitamin D are also important antioxidants to maintain healthy eyes. The daily recommended intake of selenium for adults is approximately 55 mcg of vitamin D is 200 International Units (IU).

19. Vegetables are a great source of vitamins and minerals and help improve the health of your eyes. Spinach and avocado are some of the most nutrient dense. They both contain vitamin A and lutein, which

are important in maintaining and restoring good vision. Tomatoes and broccoli are both chock full of vitamin C. Salmon and eggs are lean sources of protein that help eyesight, too. Both are also rich sources of vitamins A and D. Salmon also has Omega-3 fatty acids, which are important for overall eye health. Other foods that are helpful at preventing eye problems are garlic and sunflower seeds. Both contain selenium, which promotes eye health.

20. Any type of polluted environment over a long period of time can contribute to vision problems, including air pollution and smog. Avoid smoking and ingesting second hand smoke because these stimulate the production of free radicals that attack your cells. Obesity causes vision problems as well, so keeping your weight under control is necessary. Lastly, people with diabetes are at high risk for vision problems so they should keep blood sugar levels under control at all times.

21. Remain hydrated. Make sure that you are drinking at least 8-10 glasses of water daily and you remain hydrated. This will

help in keeping the progress of vision problems at bay. Also avoid carbonated drinks, if you feel like taking something while having lunch don't fall for carbonated drinks, prepare in advance and get a water bottle.

22. Understand the eye and the lens. A good understanding of the eye is also needed to prevent and control it's issue. See this image of the human eye.

23. Keep eyes relaxed. It is important to keep the eyes relaxed so that they get the time to heal themselves, make sure you do not spend too much time on gadgets like I-phone, tablets, Computers, Television, Video games, if you are spending a lot of time then maintain discipline and say no to such activities.

24. Salt intake. Lower the salt intake to as much as possible. Watch out for salty chips and salty packaged food. Salt has been found in some studies to cause progression of eye problems.

25. Cineraria Maritma is very effective for Cataract and is a treatment of choice in India for early cataract patients.

26. Vision problems are also known to be caused due to bad humour, if you consistently remain in bad humour you are at high risk from vision problems and even other diseases.

27. Watch a comedy channel. Notice the timings of comedy tv programs and take time out to watch them regularly.

28. Fresh pineapple juice, carrot juice helps the eyes and vision tremendously. Make it a point to consume freshly squeezed juices regularly.

13 YOUR DAILY REGIMEN

Following the daily regimen presented below will help you to stop the progression of your vision problems. The more number of points you follow daily the better.

1. Drink 8-10 glasses of water daily.

2. Take a morning or evening walk.

3. Consume a very high Vitamin C diet more than 200% daily Vitamin C quota.

4. Wash your eyes multiple times a day, for better results use an eye-cup.

5. Keep your eyes strain free.

6. Remain stress free and in good humour all day, if you can't try to find ways in which you can reduce your stress.

7. Eat several portions of fresh fruits, vegetables and juices.

8. Consume a low sugar and low salt diet. Avoid coffee, tea and dairy products.

9. Exercise daily.

10. Be cautious with drugs which have listed vision problems in their side effects.

11. Exercise your eye balls by moving them from side to side, up and down and holding the head steady.

12. Daily perform Pranayam exercises.

13. Do not allow sunrays to fall on your eye balls. Use a cap if you must go in sunlight.

14. Do not directly look at the sun, and use UV Blocking glasses.

Ending Note

Thank you for reading this book. I am sure if you follow the advice in this book you will maintain good vision and even restore your vision to a certain extent. I request all readers to leave a positive rating for the book accentuating the positives and helping other readers find this resource and acknowledging the efforts of the writer. This book has been self published on CreateSpace with no editors and with very limited budget so you would hopefully ignore some errors in the book related to grammar or spellings.

Thank You!